RECI

INGREDIENTS:

___

DIRECTIONS:

___

USES:

___

RECIPE:

INGREDIENTS:

DIRECTIONS:

USES:

RECIPE:

INGREDIENTS:

_____

_____

_____

_____

_____

_____

_____

_____

_____

_____

_____

DIRECTIONS:

_____

_____

_____

_____

_____

_____

_____

_____

_____

USES:

_____

_____

RECIPE:

INGREDIENTS:

DIRECTIONS:

USES:

RECIPE:

INGREDIENTS:

_____

_____

_____

_____

_____

_____

_____

_____

DIRECTIONS:

_____

_____

_____

_____

_____

_____

_____

_____

USES:

_____

_____

RECIPE:

_____

INGREDIENTS:

_____
_____
_____
_____
_____
_____
_____
_____

DIRECTIONS:

_____
_____
_____
_____
_____
_____
_____
_____

USES:

_____
_____

RECIPE:

INGREDIENTS:

DIRECTIONS:

USES:

RECIPE:

INGREDIENTS:

DIRECTIONS:

USES:

RECIPE:

INGREDIENTS:

DIRECTIONS:

USES:

RECIPE:

INGREDIENTS:

DIRECTIONS:

USES:

RECIPE:

INGREDIENTS:

_____

_____

_____

_____

_____

_____

_____

_____

DIRECTIONS:

_____

_____

_____

_____

_____

_____

_____

USES:

_____

_____

RECIPE:

INGREDIENTS:

DIRECTIONS:

USES:

RECIPE: _____

INGREDIENTS:

_____

_____

_____

_____

_____

_____

_____

_____

_____

DIRECTIONS:

_____

_____

_____

_____

_____

_____

_____

_____

USES:

_____

_____

RECIPE:

INGREDIENTS:

_____
_____
_____
_____
_____
_____
_____

DIRECTIONS:

_____
_____
_____
_____
_____
_____
_____
_____

USES:

_____
_____

RECIPE:

INGREDIENTS:

DIRECTIONS:

USES:

RECIPE:

INGREDIENTS:

DIRECTIONS:

USES:

RECIPE:

INGREDIENTS:

DIRECTIONS:

USES:

RECIPE:

INGREDIENTS:

_____

_____

_____

_____

_____

_____

_____

DIRECTIONS:

_____

_____

_____

_____

_____

_____

_____

USES:

_____

_____

RECIPE:

INGREDIENTS:

_____

_____

_____

_____

_____

_____

_____

_____

_____

DIRECTIONS:

_____

_____

_____

_____

_____

_____

_____

_____

USES:

_____

_____

RECIPE:

INGREDIENTS:

_____

_____

_____

_____

_____

_____

_____

DIRECTIONS:

_____

_____

_____

_____

_____

_____

_____

USES:

_____

_____

RECIPE: _____

INGREDIENTS:

_____
_____
_____
_____
_____
_____
_____
_____

DIRECTIONS:

_____
_____
_____
_____
_____
_____
_____
_____

USES:

_____
_____

RECIPE:

INGREDIENTS:

_____

_____

_____

_____

_____

_____

_____

_____

DIRECTIONS:

_____

_____

_____

_____

_____

_____

_____

_____

USES:

_____

_____

RECIPE:

INGREDIENTS:

DIRECTIONS:

USES:

RECIPE:

INGREDIENTS:

DIRECTIONS:

USES:

RECIPE:

INGREDIENTS:

DIRECTIONS:

USES:

RECIPE:

INGREDIENTS:

_____
_____
_____
_____
_____
_____
_____
_____

DIRECTIONS:

_____
_____
_____
_____
_____
_____
_____
_____

USES:

_____
_____

RECIPE:

INGREDIENTS:

DIRECTIONS:

USES:

RECIPE:

INGREDIENTS:

DIRECTIONS:

USES:

RECIPE: _____

INGREDIENTS: _____

_____

_____

_____

_____

_____

_____

_____

DIRECTIONS: _____

_____

_____

_____

_____

_____

_____

_____

USES: _____

_____

_____

RECIPE:

INGREDIENTS:

DIRECTIONS:

USES:

RECIPE: _____

INGREDIENTS:

_____
_____
_____
_____
_____
_____
_____
_____

DIRECTIONS:

_____
_____
_____
_____
_____
_____
_____
_____

USES:

_____
_____

RECIPE:

INGREDIENTS:

DIRECTIONS:

USES:

RECIPE: _____

INGREDIENTS: _____
_____
_____
_____
_____
_____
_____
_____

DIRECTIONS: _____
_____
_____
_____
_____
_____
_____
_____
_____

USES: _____
_____
_____

RECIPE:

INGREDIENTS:

DIRECTIONS:

USES:

RECIPE:

_____

INGREDIENTS:

_____
_____
_____
_____
_____
_____
_____
_____

DIRECTIONS:

_____
_____
_____
_____
_____
_____
_____
_____

USES:

_____
_____
_____

RECIPE:

INGREDIENTS:

DIRECTIONS:

USES:

RECIPE: _____

INGREDIENTS: _____

_____

_____

_____

_____

_____

_____

_____

_____

DIRECTIONS: _____

_____

_____

_____

_____

_____

_____

_____

_____

USES: _____

_____

_____

RECIPE:

INGREDIENTS:

DIRECTIONS:

USES:

RECIPE:

INGREDIENTS:

DIRECTIONS:

USES:

RECIPE:

INGREDIENTS:

DIRECTIONS:

USES:

RECIPE:

INGREDIENTS:

DIRECTIONS:

USES:

RECIPE:

INGREDIENTS:

DIRECTIONS:

USES:

RECIPE:

INGREDIENTS:

DIRECTIONS:

USES:

RECIPE:

INGREDIENTS:

DIRECTIONS:

USES:

RECIPE:

INGREDIENTS:

DIRECTIONS:

USES:

RECIPE:

INGREDIENTS:

DIRECTIONS:

USES:

RECIPE:

INGREDIENTS:

DIRECTIONS:

USES:

RECIPE:

INGREDIENTS:

DIRECTIONS:

USES:

RECIPE:

INGREDIENTS:

DIRECTIONS:

USES:

RECIPE:

INGREDIENTS:

DIRECTIONS:

USES:

RECIPE: _____

INGREDIENTS:

_____

_____

_____

_____

_____

_____

_____

_____

DIRECTIONS:

_____

_____

_____

_____

_____

_____

_____

_____

USES:

_____

_____

RECIPE:

INGREDIENTS:

DIRECTIONS:

USES:

RECIPE:

INGREDIENTS:

DIRECTIONS:

USES:

RECIPE: _____

INGREDIENTS: _____
_____
_____
_____
_____
_____
_____
_____
_____

DIRECTIONS: _____
_____
_____
_____
_____
_____
_____
_____

USES: _____
_____
_____

RECIPE:

INGREDIENTS:

DIRECTIONS:

USES:

RECIPE:

INGREDIENTS:

DIRECTIONS:

USES:

RECIPE:

INGREDIENTS:

DIRECTIONS:

USES:

RECIPE:

INGREDIENTS:

DIRECTIONS:

USES:

RECIPE:

INGREDIENTS:

DIRECTIONS:

USES:

RECIPE:

INGREDIENTS:

DIRECTIONS:

USES:

RECIPE:

INGREDIENTS:

DIRECTIONS:

USES:

RECIPE:

INGREDIENTS:

DIRECTIONS:

USES:

RECIPE: _____

INGREDIENTS:
_____
_____
_____
_____
_____
_____
_____
_____
_____

DIRECTIONS:
_____
_____
_____
_____
_____
_____
_____
_____
_____

USES:
_____
_____

RECIPE:

INGREDIENTS:

DIRECTIONS:

USES:

RECIPE:

INGREDIENTS:

DIRECTIONS:

USES:

RECIPE:

INGREDIENTS:

_____

_____

_____

_____

_____

_____

_____

DIRECTIONS:

_____

_____

_____

_____

_____

_____

_____

USES:

_____

_____

RECIPE:

INGREDIENTS:

DIRECTIONS:

USES:

RECIPE: _____

INGREDIENTS:

_____
_____
_____
_____
_____
_____
_____

DIRECTIONS:

_____
_____
_____
_____
_____
_____
_____

USES:

_____
_____

RECIPE:

INGREDIENTS:

DIRECTIONS:

USES:

RECIPE:

INGREDIENTS:

DIRECTIONS:

USES:

RECIPE:

INGREDIENTS:

DIRECTIONS:

USES:

RECIPE:

INGREDIENTS:

DIRECTIONS:

USES:

RECIPE:

INGREDIENTS:

DIRECTIONS:

USES:

RECIPE:

INGREDIENTS:

DIRECTIONS:

USES:

RECIPE:

INGREDIENTS:

DIRECTIONS:

USES:

RECIPE:

INGREDIENTS:

DIRECTIONS:

USES:

RECIPE:

INGREDIENTS:

DIRECTIONS:

USES:

RECIPE:

INGREDIENTS:

DIRECTIONS:

USES:

RECIPE:

INGREDIENTS:

DIRECTIONS:

USES:

RECIPE:

INGREDIENTS:

DIRECTIONS:

USES:

RECIPE: _____

INGREDIENTS:

_____

_____

_____

_____

_____

_____

_____

_____

_____

DIRECTIONS:

_____

_____

_____

_____

_____

_____

_____

_____

USES:

_____

_____

_____

RECIPE: _____

INGREDIENTS:

_____
_____
_____
_____
_____
_____
_____

DIRECTIONS:

_____
_____
_____
_____
_____
_____
_____

USES:

_____
_____

RECIPE:

INGREDIENTS:

DIRECTIONS:

USES:

RECIPE:

INGREDIENTS:

DIRECTIONS:

USES:

RECIPE:

INGREDIENTS:

DIRECTIONS:

USES:

RECIPE:

INGREDIENTS:

DIRECTIONS:

USES:

RECIPE:

INGREDIENTS:

DIRECTIONS:

USES:

RECIPE:

INGREDIENTS:

DIRECTIONS:

USES:

RECIPE:

INGREDIENTS:

DIRECTIONS:

USES:

RECIPE:

INGREDIENTS:

DIRECTIONS:

USES:

RECIPE:

INGREDIENTS:

DIRECTIONS:

USES:

RECIPE:

INGREDIENTS:

DIRECTIONS:

USES:

RECIPE:

INGREDIENTS:

DIRECTIONS:

USES:

RECIPE:

INGREDIENTS:

DIRECTIONS:

USES:

RECIPE:

INGREDIENTS:

DIRECTIONS:

USES:

RECIPE:

_____

INGREDIENTS:

_____
_____
_____
_____
_____
_____
_____
_____

DIRECTIONS:

_____
_____
_____
_____
_____
_____
_____

USES:

_____
_____

RECIPE:

INGREDIENTS:

DIRECTIONS:

USES:

RECIPE: _____

INGREDIENTS:

_____
_____
_____
_____
_____
_____
_____

DIRECTIONS:

_____
_____
_____
_____
_____
_____
_____

USES:

_____
_____

RECIPE:

INGREDIENTS:

DIRECTIONS:

USES:

RECIPE:

INGREDIENTS:

DIRECTIONS:

USES:

Made in the USA
Columbia, SC
13 October 2020